Live Better aromatherapy

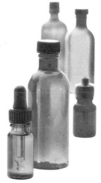

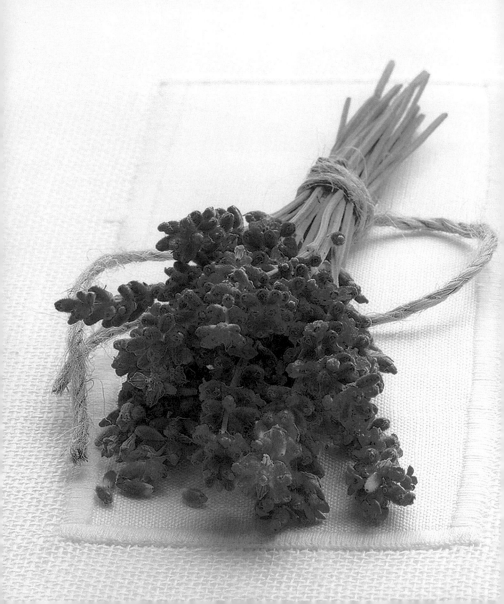

Live Better aromatherapy

Remedies and inspirations for well-being

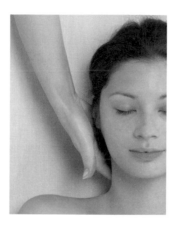

Jennie Harding

DUNCAN BAIRD PUBLISHERS

LONDON

Live Better: Aromatherapy
Jennie Harding

For my mother Sonja, whose love and light always inspires me.

First published in the United Kingdom
and Ireland in 2006 by
Duncan Baird Publishers Ltd
Sixth Floor
Castle House
75–76 Wells Street
London W1T 3QH

Conceived, created and designed by
Duncan Baird Publishers Ltd
Copyright © Duncan Baird Publishers 2006
Text copyright © Jennie Harding 2006
Commissioned photography copyright © Duncan Baird
Publishers 2006
For copyright of agency photographs see p.128, which is to
be regarded as an extension of this copyright.

Managing Designer: Manisha Patel
Designer: Justin Ford
Managing Editor: Grace Cheetham
Editor: Zoë Stone
Picture Research: Susannah Stone
Commissioned Photography: William Lingwood

British Library Cataloguing-in-Publication Data:
A CIP record for this book is available from the
British Library.

ISBN-10: 1-84483-294-5
ISBN-13: 9-781844-832941

10 9 8 7 6 5 4 3 2 1

Typeset in Filosofia and Son Kern
Colour reproduction by Scanhouse, Malaysia
Printed in Malaysia by Imago

Publisher's note

Before following any advice or practice suggested in
this book, it is recommended that you consult a
medical practitioner as to its suitability, especially if
you suffer from any health problems or special
conditions, or if you are pregnant. The publishers,
author and photographers cannot accept any
responsibility for any injuries or damage incurred
as a result of using any of the therapeutic methods
described or mentioned here.

Note on measurements

The aromatherapy blends contained in this book are
measured in teaspoons and tablespoons: 1 teaspoon
is 5ml and 1 tablespoon is 15ml.

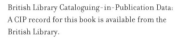

contents

Introduction

Welcome to *Live Better: Aromatherapy* — a journey into a wonderful perfumed world. This book shows you how to use delightful natural fragrances called essential oils, the tools of aromatherapy. You will learn how to relax, uplift or transform your mind, as well as help your body to feel more at ease if you are under stress.

Aromatherapy has become very popular in recent years, but many people are still not quite sure what aromatherapy actually is or how it works. This book shows you clearly, safely and creatively how to experience the art of aromatherapy yourself and choose natural essential oils to fragrance your environment, perfume your bath or massage into your skin so you experience their effects directly. Aromatherapy can have an impact on mood, feelings and emotions, as well as physical problems such as muscular aches and pains. Read on to discover how powerful your sense of smell is, and how you can work with it using aromatherapy techniques to help rebalance and re-energize both mind and body.

Imagine you are walking through a park or a garden on a warm summer's day and you see a spectacular rose bush covered with heavy pink blooms. What is your reaction? You may be attracted by the shape of the flowers, or their exact shade of pink, but you cannot experience the rose directly without burying your face in those soft, cool petals so the sweet, honey-like, lemony aroma fills your nose. You breathe in, you sigh, your senses are alert and filled with the fragrance. Perhaps it recalls something to you – a memory, a place, a time. Maybe there is a feeling attached to that memory. Perhaps the scent of the rose helps you to release an emotion, to breathe deeply and relax, to feel at peace.

This is the essence of aromatherapy – the experience of a fragrance, its effect on the senses, a change in mood. However, therapeutically we take that experience further, because we also make practical use of the concentrated fragrance of the oil: by applying it to the body we achieve physical effects as well. This book shows you how to do all this for yourself easily and effectively, so that aromatherapy can make a real difference to your life.

origins and basics

In this chapter we will explore more closely what aromatherapy actually is and how it works. This is important because, as you start to use aromatherapy, you will notice physical and mental effects: changes you sense through your skin and your breathing, impacting on your moods. It helps to understand how and why these changes are happening; that way you can really appreciate the beneficial effects of essential oils and aromatherapy on your body and your mind.

We will also look at how aromatherapy has evolved over the years. The use of aromatic plants is nothing new: these fragrances have fascinated humankind for thousands of years. Ancient peoples used natural aromas to make incense, medicines, cosmetics and fragrances, and they considered the plants which produced them to have links to the spiritual world, a belief which persists in certain cultures today.

Modern aromatherapy reinterprets the subtle aspects of these fragrances, focusing on the mental effects and therapeutic benefits of essential oils. The feeling of lightness and a happier, more peaceful state of mind are among these benefits, making aromatherapy a wonderful antidote to the pressures of modern life. Stress is an ever-increasing part of our lives, and this can only mean that aromatherapy is more relevant today than ever before.

WHAT IS AROMATHERAPY?

A growing contemporary interest in aromatherapy has meant that it has come to mean different things to different people. To many professional aromatherapy practitioners, aromatherapy is a gentle art that can have profound effects on body and mind. To botanists and biochemistry experts, essential oils are complex packages of molecules. To those with a scientific approach, aromatherapy is the subtle application of bio-active ingredients, and to a perfumer essential oils are the building blocks of fragrances. Aromatherapy is all of these things – it reflects aspects of art and science, perfume and psychology, biochemistry and botany.

More simply, aromatherapy can be split into two words – "aroma" and "therapy". "Aroma" clearly indicates a link to the sense of smell, which picks up and interprets chemical messages. "Therapy" implies that the fragrance is applied to someone to achieve a particular beneficial effect. In the next few pages we will look at these aspects in more detail.

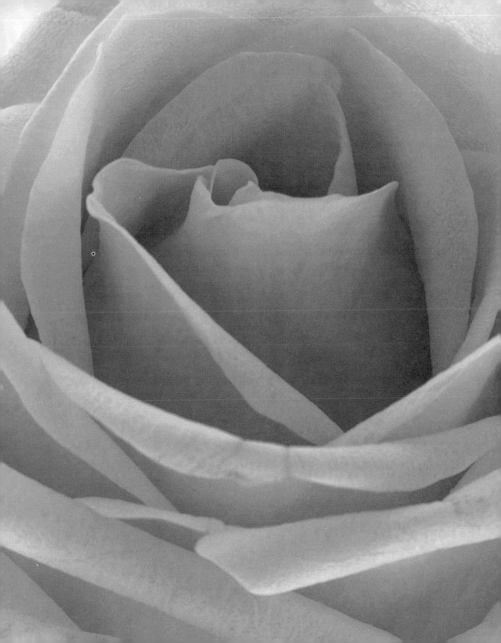

THE POWER OF SMELL

We are often unaware of our sense of smell: many people only notice it when it is temporarily absent. For example, during a heavy cold we notice that everything feels remote, and that food has no taste. This is because 80 percent of what we taste comes from our sense of smell; only 20 percent comes from the tongue. If someone loses their sense of smell permanently, this can actually cause severe depression. Why? Because we rely very deeply on the sense of smell to add richness and vitality to our experience of the world around us.

Smells register via the nose as we breathe, travelling up the nostrils and triggering nerve impulses which fire instantly into the brain. Thousands of these reactions occur daily, even when we are asleep. Smells have a strong influence on our well-being because they affect areas inside the brain linked to moods, emotions or feelings, as well as chemical balances in the body. So, aromas which make you feel mentally calm also trigger internal chemical changes, relaxing your body.

Fragrances which are more revitalizing stimulate the brain, wake you up and give you a feeling of energy.

Some impulses received by the sense of smell affect areas deep inside the brain which are beyond conscious awareness; very often reactions to smells are expressed as non-verbal sounds such as "mmmm" or "urgh!". These show that our responses to smells are instinctive, a simple "like" or "dislike". This is evident in small children who automatically reach toward what smells good and move abruptly away from what smells bad.

In adults, strong instinctive responses to aromas usually stem from associated memories. The French writer Marcel Proust's epic novel *A la recherche du temps perdu* (In Search of Lost Time) centres on one smell – a madeleine cake dipped in lime-flower tea – which triggers powerful, detailed memories of his early life.

If you have never before paid much attention to your sense of smell, it is fun to start observing it more closely. For example, simply go outside and walk about for 20 minutes, to see how many scents you detect. You may be surprised by the number of aromas there are!

THERAPEUTIC APPLICATION

The second part of the word aromatherapy implies a kind of action. How do we apply these special natural fragrances? Well, there are two pathways for essential oils to enter the human body.

First, there is the avenue provided by breathing and the lungs. We have just explored the sense of smell via the nose, but of course we also breathe through the mouth. Essential oils can travel through the mouth into the passageways of the respiratory tract as far as the lungs. Pungent oils such as Eucalyptus are a good example of this at work; if you have a cold, or a blocked nose, inhaling such a powerful aroma will open up the respiratory passages, improving breathing and also helping to loosen mucus, making it easier to cough.

The second avenue of entry is via the skin. The skin has many layers; overlapping cells like microscopic roof tiles on the surface, and deeper layers richly supplied with blood vessels, nerves, sweat glands and oil glands. Taking baths with essential oils as well as using massage brings these oils into direct contact with your skin. The warmth of bath water or the friction heat generated by massage helps the tiny essential oils molecules to pass through the top layer of the skin and enter the bloodstream. From there they can be used by the body where needed, passing out of the system via the kidneys. Massaging an aching back with Rosemary, for example, will give a feeling of warmth to the muscles, improving local blood supply and easing away stiffness.

Essential oils fall into different groups according to what they do. Calming oils such as Lavender or Orange Blossom help to ease physical pain, soothing aching muscles or headaches, and have a sedative effect on body and mind. Pungent oils such as Black Pepper or Cardamon have an energizing effect, warming poor circulation, producing a feeing of physical vitality. Fresh oils such as Peppermint or Rosemary are stimulating, cleansing the body and removing toxins as well as improving concentration. Citrus aromas such as Lemon or Mandarin aid the flow of digestive juices, tonifying the system; they also help combat depression.

The infinite has written its name on the heavens in
shinning stars, and on the earth in tender flowers.

JEAN PAUL RICHTER

(1763 – 1825)

Our highest assurance of the goodness of providence
seems to me to rest in the flowers.

SIR ARTHUR CONAN DOYLE

(1859 – 1930)

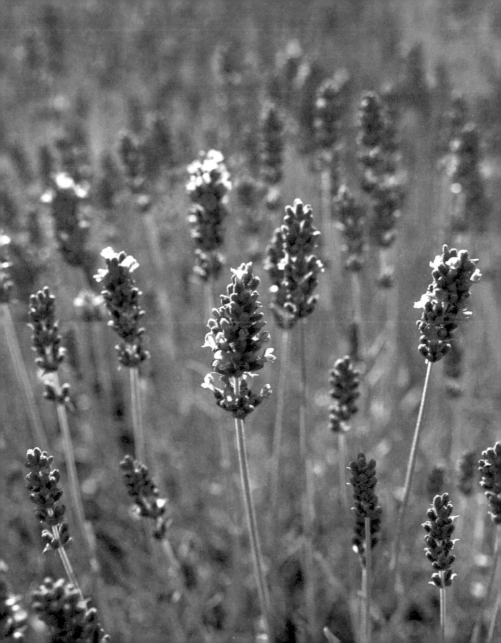

ANCIENT AROMATIC HISTORY

No one knows exactly how or when our ancestors first became interested in aromatic plants, but archaeological evidence points to very early use. In excavations of prehistoric burials in Iraq, the remains of wreaths made from plants have been identified. Pollen grains show that aromatic species were preferred, ones which still grow in the region today.

In early civilizations such as those of Mesopotamia 3–4,000 years ago, herbs and spices were used to treat disease. The role of the healer was to purify the patient's body and mind, expelling evil spirits; aromatics were used to fumigate the area, creating a healing space around the sick person to cleanse them and restore balance. This practice persists around the world today. For example, in Peru, special practitioners called *curanderas* (women) and *curanderos* (men) use aromatic herbs as incense and as infusions to heal disease.

In ancient Egypt, the boundary between priest and healer did not exist. At Abydos on the Nile, excavations of the healing temple of Osiris revealed a series of underground rooms, each with a hole in the ceiling. Inscriptions explain that patients would consult the priests and be instructed to sleep in one of the chambers overnight. Incense would be burned over the sleeping patient, and in the morning the priests would interpret the patient's dreams, thereby unlocking the source of their sickness. The fragrance was the key to the patient's unconscious mind.

Aromas also defined status in the ancient world; kings, queens and potentates demonstrated their wealth by being lavishly perfumed. Wreaths of aromatic plants such as mint and myrtle adorned banqueting tables, and guests would wear garlands of scented flowers and herbs to aid digestion. Conical hats impregnated with aromas such as frankincense were sometimes worn at ancient Egyptian feasts so perfume melted over the wearer during the meal! In ancient Greece and Rome, wealthy men and women had themselves perfumed in layers – different fragrances were applied to different parts of their bodies, creating waves of scent as they walked.

THE SPLENDOUR OF EGYPT

When the grave of the pharaoh Tutankhamun was excavated, each of the many coffins was covered with astonishing wreaths of aromatic flowers and herbs. Fortunately a botanist photographed and identified the plants used before they fell into dust. The flowers included species of lotus, long revered as a sacred bloom, as well as lilies. Jars of ointment containing frankincense, myrrh, spikenard and cassia could still be faintly smelled after so many years in the dark.

To the ancient Egyptians, aromatics were often a link to the gods. They were burned as incense on altars and used to anoint the pharaoh in life, as well as embalm him in death. Ingredients such as cedarwood and frankincense were also used to make cosmetic preparations and perfumes. A famous fragrance recipe of 16 ingredients called "kyphi" survives, said to brighten dreams and relieve anxiety. This ancient use of fragrance to ease anxiety is a parallel with modern aromatherapy's use of essential oils to uplift moods.

OTHER ANCIENT AROMATIC CIVILIZATIONS

Many other cultures have persisting ancient traditions of aromatic use. These uses may be linked to medicine, perfumery, cosmetics or religious ceremony. Often the same plant finds its way into all of these – for example, in India, patchouli leaves are used to cure skin problems, as the basis for incense, as a perfume ingredient and to repel moths.

India has an aromatic tradition that dates back thousands of years. The exotic aroma of sandalwood is distilled from the inner wood of this special tree and is used as a cosmetic and perfume ingredient and in the making of incense; it is burned at Hindu burials to purify the spirits of the deceased. Statues of many gods are washed daily and anointed with scented oils, wreathed in flowers and purified with incense. Ayurveda, the traditional medicine of India, makes extensive use of herbs, spices and essential oils such as Cardamom to fight infection and rebalance the body and mind.

Chinese aromatic tradition used powdered cinnamon and cassia in the making of incense around 4,000 years ago. China's herbal medicine tradition is also very ancient, relying on a whole range of different plant ingredients such as angelica and camphor. A Chinese herbalist today will know the properties of hundreds of individual aromatic herbs and spices.

The ancient Arab culture brought many aromatics to Western Europe; its traders opened up routes to the East, allowing plants such as the orange tree and the rose to spread across the globe. The Arabs are credited with discovering distillation, which uses heat to extract essential oils from aromatic material. Abu Ibn Sina, or Avicenna (980–1037), was a remarkable physician, philosopher and scientist who created a simple form of this technique.

Some 2,000 years later, distillation techniques still produce most essential oils used in aromatherapy. Essential oils are produced worldwide, both in a small way, using very simple stills, and on a large commercial scale with high-tech equipment.

MODERN AROMATHERAPY

The French perfume chemist R.M. Gattefosse created the word "aromathérapie" in the 1930s after applying some Lavender essential oil to a burn on his hand. He was astonished at the speed with which it healed, and went on to publish a book highlighting the healing potential of essential oils, which became a classic.

Until that time, essential oils had been in and out of popular use. In the 16th and 17th centuries, improvements in distillation technology in Germany and Switzerland made essential oils more widely available. Aromatic spices such as cloves, cinnamon and nutmeg were used as antiseptics during the plague.

However, in the 17th and 18th centuries, rising interest in chemical drugs in Western Europe lead to a decline in the medicinal use of herbs and essential oils, although the perfumery industry in southern France continued with large-scale distillation of lavender and rose into the 19th century. One French report noted that perfumery workers were far less likely to suffer from tuberculosis, but no one at the time realized that exposure to essential oils was the key protective factor.

In the 20th century, in France, Gattefosse and other pioneers such as Dr Jean Valnet, a scientist interested in the antiseptic powers of essential oils, and Marguerite Maury, who put forward the idea of using massage to administer oils, paved the way for modern aroma-therapy. In the UK, Robert Tisserand's book *The Art of Aromatherapy* (1975) triggered an explosion of interest in the subject leading to its development in public practice.

Today, aromatherapy has spread around the world. It is most popular in English-speaking countries. There is rapidly growing interest in the Far East and South America, and it is used in European countries, often under the guise of beauty therapy. The US and UK style differs from the more aesthetic approach; in a professional treatment, three essential oils are chosen and diluted in vegetable oil, making a blend which is then massaged all over the body. The choice of essential oils is based on the client's physical and emotional state, to help them feel relaxed and revitalized.

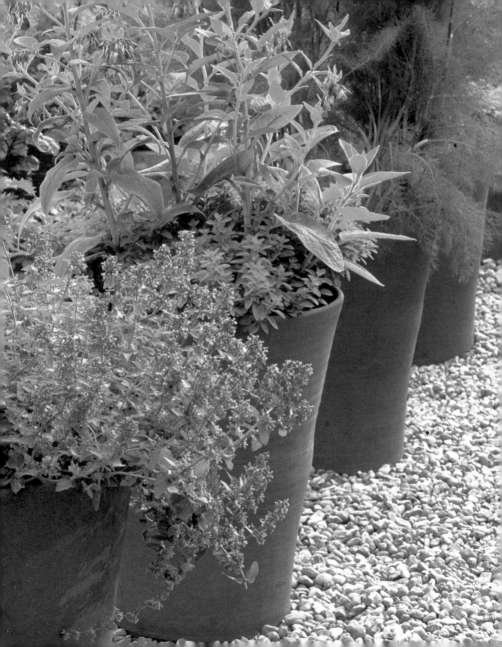

He who has health has hope; and he who has hope
has everything.

ARABIC PROVERB

The garden is the poor man's apothecary.

GERMAN PROVERB

WHAT AROMATHERAPY CAN DO FOR YOU

Regular use of essential oils can greatly enhance your well-being, helping you to ward off stress and deal with the pressures of modern life.

Essential oils can make a real difference to your energy levels; you can choose to use revitalizing oils if you need to feel re-energized, or relaxing oils if you need to rest and be at ease. Building an aromatic bath into your evening routine can help improve your sleep patterns and give you better quality rest.

You can vaporize essential oils and use them in the home, or even at work, to help improve your environment. As we have already seen, some oils can help keep your mind alert and improve your concentration.

Using essential oils in baths, inhalations and massage can improve the function of your immune system – helping you to recover quickly from illness, as well as building your resistance to infections such as colds and flu. This is particularly helpful in the winter. See Chapter 3 for some fantastic immune-boosting oils.

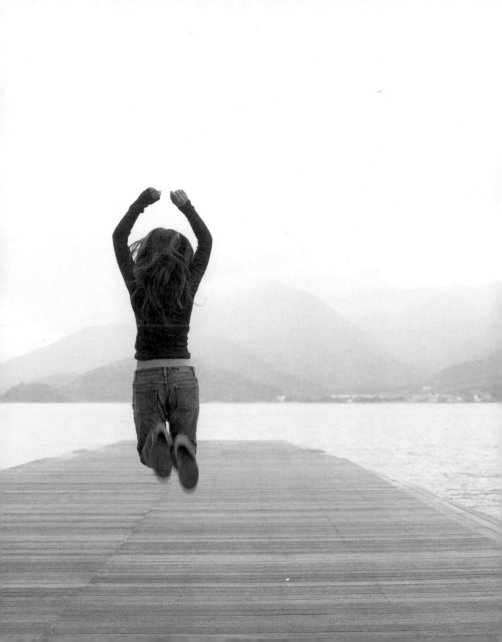

HOW TO USE THIS BOOK

You can easily practise aromatherapy on yourself at home – this book shows you how. In the following chapter you will find clear and detailed guidelines on how to use essential oils practically and safely. It's important to read all this information carefully and make sure you understand it; that way you will be using aromatherapy effectively right from the start. Chapter 3 presents detailed profiles of the top 20 essential oils, organized according to the moods they produce – choose between oils to relax, inspire, uplift or revitalize.

The best way to use this book is to read it thoroughly, taking in the images and inspirations as well as the practical information and the individual essential oil profiles. These may well prompt you to buy some oils to try at home. When you do, take care to observe the tips for buying and storing oils on pages 44–6.

If you decide you want to use the oils in massage, it is worth investing in a more detailed book on aromatherapy massage to guide you through the routines.

It is easy enough to rub the oils into the skin, but learning some actual massage techniques can be particularly effective, because the power of therapeutic touch complements perfectly the use of essential oils.

When it comes to selecting and buying essential oils, it really is a matter of personal preference. But when people ask "What should my basic kit include?" I usually suggest starting with the familiar oil Lavender, which is useful for everything from first aid to promoting sleep. I then go on to include some other common, useful oils such as Peppermint for nausea and headaches or Rosemary for aching muscles. All the most common oils are profiled in this book. Also covered are oils with more specific properties and uses, which you will most likely purchase as the need arises.

Getting used to the intensity of essential oils takes time. Any essential oil is approximately a hundred times more concentrated in its bottled form than the aroma was in the original plant. This is why it's best to use familiar fragrances to begin with. Start with five or six oils and get to know them before you add to your collection.

Look in the perfumes of flowers and of Nature for peace
of mind and joy of life.

WANG WEI

(8TH CENTURY CE)

Ointment and perfume rejoice the heart.

PROVERBS 27:9

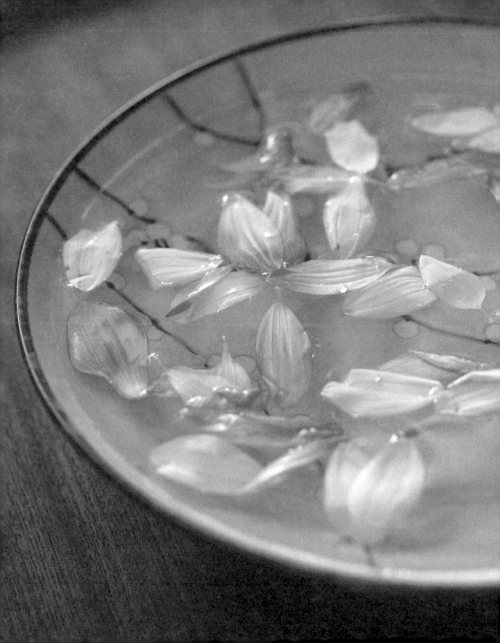

Chapter Two

aromatherapy
know-how

This chapter tells you all you need to know to practise aromatherapy safely and appropriately, as well as creatively, to obtain maximum benefit for health and well-being.

You will discover ways of using essential oils at home – from baths and inhalations to vaporizers and massages. Some of these methods require you to purchase some basic equipment, but there are many suitable outlets for you to do so.

Safety guidelines regarding essential oils are very important. Aromatherapy uses ingredients that are 100 percent natural; however, these concentrated substances need to be used in an informed way. Essential oils must be used carefully on older people, babies, children and people with skin problems. Always follow the guidelines given on page 47.

You will also find easy-to-follow, practical information on how to make up your aromatherapy blends. Teaspoons and tablespoons are used throughout: 1 teaspoon measures 5ml and 1 tablespoon measures 15 ml. There is also advice on buying and storing your essential oils.

Enjoy the fun of learning how to use essential oils easily and effectively for yourself, family and friends.

AROMATHERAPY BATHS

An aromatherapy bath is a luxurious treat. Preparing the space and taking at least 20 minutes to soak will allow the aromas of your chosen oils to delight your senses. As you bathe, tiny micro-droplets of essential oil will caress your body and condition your skin.

Run your bath to a comfortably warm temperature. It's a good idea to add about 2 teaspoons unfragranced bath foam or 2 tablespoons full-cream milk, to soften the water and protect your skin against any reactions.

Now for the essential oils. You will notice in the following suggestions how little oil you need. Please don't be tempted to add more, as the amounts given are quite enough to create a gorgeous bath treatment.

For a relaxing, skin-soothing soak, try 3 drops Lavender and 3 drops Rosewood. Another suggestion is 3 drops Sandalwood, 3 drops Frankincense, for a calming, woody aroma. If you are feeling low, try 2 drops Ylang Ylang and 4 drops Sweet Orange to lift your mood.

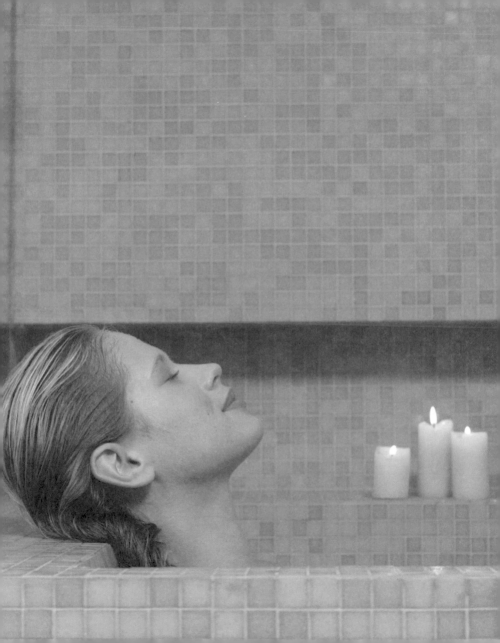

AROMATHERAPY VAPORIZERS

Using a vaporizer is a very good way to experience the simple power of aromatherapy without contact with the skin. This method is especially useful for small children and the elderly, who can be more sensitive to the effects of direct contact with essential oils (see page 47).

A vaporizer is a piece of equipment that spreads an aroma through a given space. There are many electrical models available from mail order suppliers and retail outlets. Some have a fan inside which gently blows the fragrance into the room, others heat up slightly to release the aroma into the air. Electrical vaporizers are very helpful to those who have problems sleeping; they can be left running quite safely overnight.

Why use a vaporizer? Your sense of smell will pick up on the essential oils, and you will notice corresponding effects. For example, the relaxing aroma of Lavender can help you to sleep; the fresh fragrance of Grapefruit enlivens your senses; pungent Peppermint can help to clear a blocked nose or ease hayfever symptoms.

Vaporizers are now being used in hospitals, schools, hotels and the workplace, because the devices bring the natural antiseptic and cleansing particles of essential oils into the atmosphere, helping to keep germs at bay. Scientific studies have also shown that using different fragrances at certain times of day can have varied effects on mood. For example, in a care home for older people, fresh citrus smells can help stimulate appetites before lunch, while relaxing Lavender gently promotes an afternoon nap.

Six drops of one or a combination of essential oils will usually provide fragrance for up to two hours. This varies with the general temperature – the warmer it is, the quicker the oils will evaporate, and the sooner you may need to replace them. Add the oils to the equipment according to the manufacturer's instructions.

Good combinations to try are: 3 drops Peppermint and 3 drops Lemon to clear the air and ease a blocked nose; 3 drops Sweet Orange and 3 drops Sandalwood to soothe and relax emotional stress; or 3 drops Myrtle and 3 drops Mandarin to lift your mood.

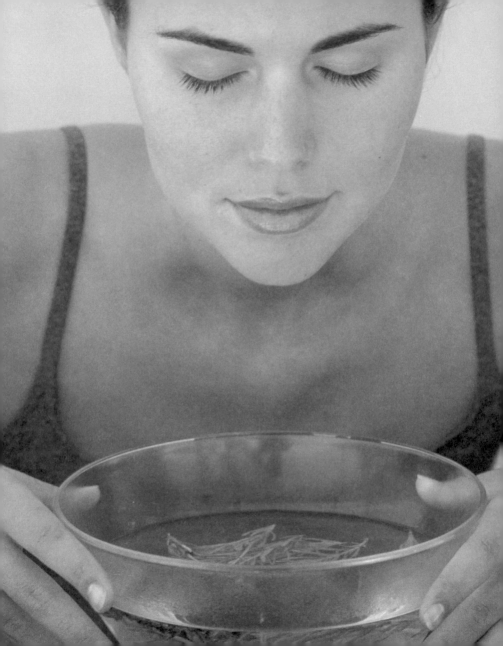

AROMATHERAPY INHALATIONS

Essential oils can have a clearing effect on the lungs through an inhalation treatment. They are particularly effective at easing respiratory problems; the oils soothe inflamed tissues, ease breathing and loosen chesty coughs as the steam carries them deep into your chest.

Inhalations are not recommended for those with asthma, mainly because inhaling steam in a confined space is uncomfortable for them. Remove glasses or contact lenses before an inhalation treatment and always supervise children carefully.

Pour about 2 litres (70fl oz) near-boiling water into a heatproof bowl. Add the essential oil. Sit with your head over the bowl, draping a towel over you to make a "tent". Lift the towel occasionally to aid breathing and inhale slowly and gently for 15 minutes.

Try 3 drops Atlas Cedarwood and 3 drops Frankincense to ease breathing; 3 drops Peppermint and 3 drops Rosemary to clear congestion; or 3 drops Cardamom and 3 drops Lemon to soothe a cough.

AROMATHERAPY MASSAGE

The practice of aromatherapy massage involves diluting essential oils in a vegetable oil so they are safe to massage into the skin. In Chapter 3 you will find many different blends to try in the essential oil profiles.

You need a good-quality vegetable oil to use as a base (carrier). Sweet almond, grapeseed and apricot kernel oils are widely available from health-food stores. (Nut allergy sufferers should use grapeseed oil only.)

Pour 4 teaspoons carrier oil into a small glass bottle or ceramic cup. Add the drops of essential oils suggested for your blend and shake or stir well.

Adding drops of essential oil to a carrier oil in the amounts given here creates a much softer and subtler aroma than oils that are undiluted. This is correct and much safer for the skin. A blend has a shelf life of up to four weeks at a temperature of 15°C (59°F).

All the blends in this book are calculated at 8 drops total essential oils to 4 teaspoons carrier oil; this is called a 2 percent dilution, suitable for normal skin.

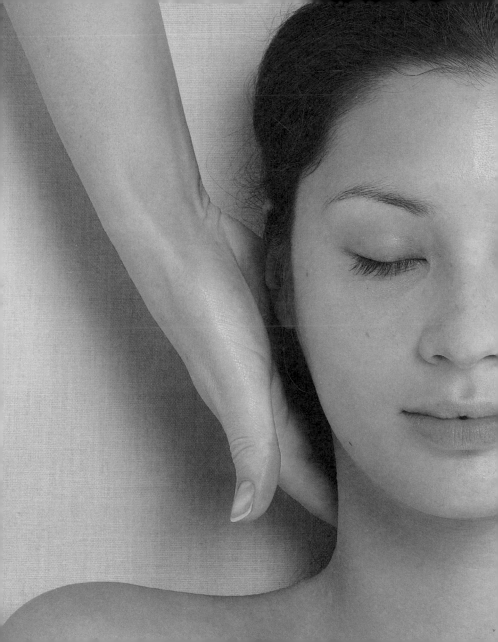

USING ESSENTIAL OILS AND CARRIER OILS

If you want the best effects from using aromatherapy, you will need to make sure you have the right tools. You will also need to make sure that you know how to take care of them properly. Collecting essential oils is fun, but you should be aware of some helpful facts before you start, so that you obtain the best possible quality materials to work with.

Buying Essential Oils and Carrier Oils

Generally, the best place to find fresh essential oils is a health-food shop where small amounts are stocked and replaced regularly. It is a good idea to ask the shop owner how often they replenish their stock.

Check where the oils are displayed: if they are sitting under hot, strong light then do not purchase them as the quality will have deteriorated and they will be less potent. Oils are best kept cool and in shade. Look for bottles with a dropper insert, which is a stopper in the neck of the bottle that only dispenses one drop at a time. This is a safety feature and helps prevent any accidental swallowing of large quantities.

There are many retail suppliers selling essential oils. If possible, try to obtain information about the company before you buy, including where they source their oils and what their company policy is concerning sustainability issues, such as Rosewood oil production. A reputable company should be able to tell you where all their oils come from and how they test them for purity.

Carrier oils are also best bought in a health-food shop. Look for "cold-pressed" oils, preferably those which are organic. They may be a little more expensive, but organic, cold-pressed carrier oils have the advantage of containing the full complement of vitamins and skin-nourishing nutrients. Cheaper carrier oils tend to be chemically refined and heat treated, which destroys the active ingredients.

Many people find it convenient to buy materials online, but make sure that you are purchasing good-quality products from a guaranteed reputable source.

Storage

Essential oils and carrier oils are natural materials with definite shelf lives that need to be observed. Once they have deteriorated they are no longer therapeutically useful and can cause skin allergies. Buy small quantities, use them fresh, then replace them – this is a good guide.

Once you open a new bottle of essential oil, the shelf life is calculated from that date. Citrus oils – Mandarin, Grapefruit and Lemon, plus Tea Tree, have a short shelf life of six months maximum at room temperature. If you store them in the refrigerator it will be a year. All other essential oils can be kept for a year at room temperature, or two years in the refrigerator.

In general, keep essential oils cool, tightly closed and in the dark. Heat, air and ultra-violet light are the main causes of deterioration, so this guideline is important.

Carrier oils can usually be stored for 6–9 months, and in the summer are best kept refrigerated. As soon as they smell sharp or musty they must be discarded.

Finally, keep all essential oils well out of the reach of children.

Aromatherapy Safety Tips

Here are some important safety tips for self-help aromatherapy. People with sensitive skin, pregnant women, older people and children aged between 3 and 10 require half the usual number of drops of essential oils in a blend: that is, 4 drops total essential oil (instead of 8) in 4 teaspoons carrier oil. This is a 1 percent dilution. Babies and infants under 3 years of age are best treated only by a qualified aromatherapist.

Essential oils should not usually be applied neat to the skin, but should always be diluted in a carrier oil for massage. Lavender is an exception (see page 57).

Keep essential oils well out of the reach of children. If any liquid is accidentally swallowed, then seek medical advice immediately.

Anyone with epilepsy or high blood pressure should avoid Rosemary as it has powerful effects on the brain and circulation. If you massage a blend containing Orange, Lemon, Mandarin or Grapefruit into the skin, avoid exposure to strong sunlight for 12 hours after application, as these oils can cause sun sensitivity.

Take the breath of the new dawn and make it part of
you. It will give you strength.

HOPI SAYING

All the flowers of all the tomorrows are in the
seeds of today.

INDIAN PROVERB

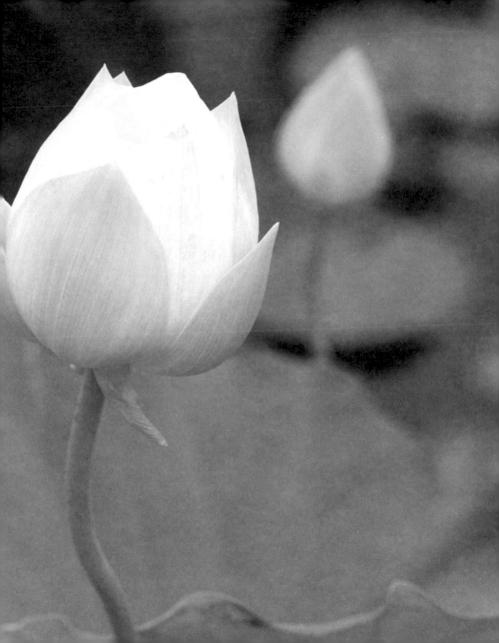

essential oil directory

In this chapter we will explore 20 of the top essential oils in detail, looking at the plants they come from and how best to use them in aromatherapy. Find out how to make soothing massage blends, purifying body scrubs and replenishing facial treatments. Learn how to create delicious fragrances for the bath and ways to make your home smell fabulous, as well as how to use essential oils to maintain your health.

The oils are organized according to the effect they have on your mind and body, and are divided into four groups: oils to help you relax, oils to inspire, oils to uplift and oils to revitalize, so you can easily pick a fragrance to suit your mood or needs.

Most essential oils are produced using steam distillation, which requires vast amounts of plant material. Citrus essential oils, such as Lemon, are obtained by expression – literally pressing oil out of the peel of the fruit. Delicate flowers, such as jasmine, require a complex process called solvent extraction, where the flowers are soaked in a chemical solvent which is then refined to produce a tiny amount of highly scented liquid, known as an absolute.

Essential oils are exquisite plant extracts that are complex and labour-intensive to produce. Enjoy experimenting with them, and let your personal collection become a palette of glorious aromas.

ESSENTIAL OILS TO RELAX

This first group of essential oils has been picked for its superb relaxing properties. These oils have a mild and soothing effect on the body and mind and are very useful for evening treatments to help you unwind from a stressful day. Relaxation is not just the physical letting go of tight muscles; it is also the releasing of tension in your thoughts. Body and mind work together, and so unlocking deep-rooted mental stress is key to achieving internal balance. These gentle essential oils envelop you in soft and soothing fragrances which can help you sleep better too, so you wake up feeling refreshed and rested.

All these oils are also particularly beneficial to women in the later stages of pregnancy. A gentle massage using large, circular strokes over the base of the lower back or a foot massage with any of these essential oils will help to calm and destress the mother-to-be. Remember that for pregnant women any blends given in the profiles only need half the stated number of drops of essential oil in the same amount of carrier oil.

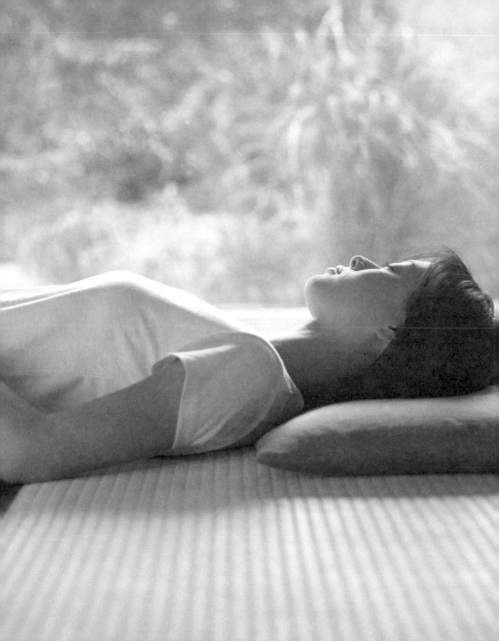

SANDALWOOD
Santalum Album

Rich, woody and sweet, the aroma of pure Sandalwood essential oil grows warmer and softer as it evaporates. The oil makes a wonderful blend because it leaves long-lasting, slightly spicy notes on the skin. It is a popular ingredient in fragrances for both men and women.

Sandalwood comes from India, where it has been used as an incense, perfume and cosmetic for at least 4,000 years. The sandalwood trees have to mature for a minimum of 30 years to allow the essential oil to develop to full saturation in the wood. Small wood chippings are used for essential oil extraction and making incense.

Sandalwood is mentally soothing and relaxing. For massage it blends extremely well with other relaxing and detoxifying oils. In 4 teaspoons carrier oil, add 4 drops Sandalwood, 2 drops Grapefruit and 2 drops Neroli (Orange Blossom) to make a beautiful refreshing aroma. It can also be use to soothe urinary problems such as cystitis: add 4–6 drops to your bath water.

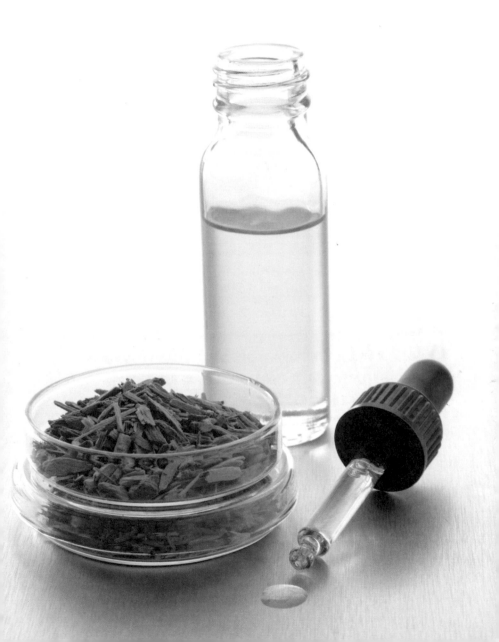

LAVENDER
Lavandula Angustifolia

Clusters of purple flowers swaying in a warm summer breeze, releasing a soft, powdery aroma into the air... lavender is a classic summer fragrance, flowery and familiar. The plant was probably introduced to the UK by the Romans. In the Middle Ages it was a favourite cure for headaches, and in the 17th century the English herbalist Nicholas Culpeper recommended it for nervous stress and tension.

Vast fields of purple lavender are also a feature of the landscape in southern France, particularly in Provence, where fine-quality essential oil has been produced for several hundred years. The oil is obtained from the flowers and stalks; the flowers add the soft, fragrant notes and the stalks the more fresh, pungent tones when the plant is distilled.

Lavender and other aromatic plants belonging to the same botanical family, such as rosemary and thyme, originated in the Mediterranean region and all thrive in a hot climate: the hottest and driest climates produce the greatest quantity of oil, with the most pungent aroma.

Lavender oil is a gentle and soothing remedy. Most essential oils should not be used neat on the skin, but Lavender is an exception: 2 drops neat on a cotton-wool pad can be applied directly to cuts, grazes, minor burns, insect bites and stings, and 2 drops on the fingertips can be applied to the forehead to help ease a headache.

In a vaporizer, Lavender can be used to cure sleeping problems. It is a good idea to start the vaporizer about 20 minutes before you go to bed, so your room is already lightly fragranced when you lie down to sleep. If you have difficulty unwinding, try using 3 drops Lavender and 3 drops Sandalwood in a warm bath before you go to bed.

In massage, Lavender is a wonderful oil to use for aches and pains and easing tight muscles. It relieves pain and cramps and helps to relax tension. Combined with circulation-stimulating oils such as Rosemary and Cardamom, it makes a superb blend for back massage. In 4 teaspoons carrier oil, add 4 drops Lavender, 2 drops Rosemary and 2 drops Cardamom.

SPECIAL LAVENDER DETOX TREATMENT

This is a spa-style treatment that can be used to treat areas such as the thighs, which can suffer from unsightly cellulite. Make up the scrub and massage oil and then use both daily for at least a week to start seeing results.

Lavender and Grapefruit Purifying Salt Scrub

In a clean glass jar pour in 8 tablespoons fine sea salt. Add 10 drops Lavender and 6 drops Grapefruit. Shake thoroughly. A small handful of the scrub rubbed into the skin while showering helps to tone problem areas. This amount will last for up to eight treatments.

Lavender and Sandalwood Massage Oil

In 4 teaspoons carrier oil, add 4 drops Lavender and 6 drops Sandalwood. Lavender is gently cleansing and Sandalwood detoxifies the body. This blend will make one full body treatment or 3–4 treatments on a local area such as the thighs. Massage the blend into the skin after the shower treatment.

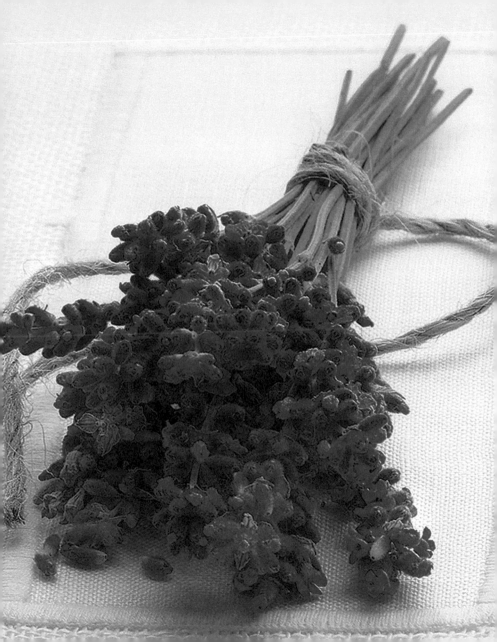

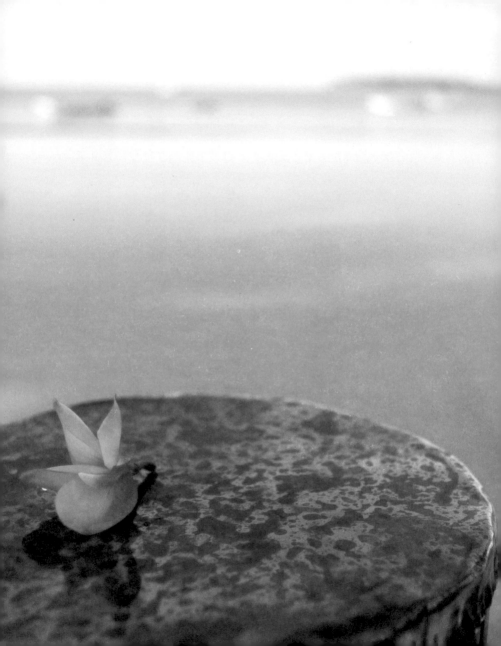

Away from the chatter of the senses, from the restless
wanderings of the mind, there is a quiet pool of
stillness. The wise call this stillness the highest state
of being. It is the place where we find unity — never to
become separate again.

THE UPANISHADS

(c1000BCE)

SWEET ORANGE
Citrus Sinensis

Deliciously sweet and filled with tangy, citrus freshness, Sweet Orange essential oil has a mouthwatering aroma. If you pare off a thin strip of fresh orange peel and turn it over, you will see the small, round sacs containing the essential oil, and you will immediately smell it – that's why grated orange zest smells so good.

Orange trees originated in China, where the peel was used to treat stomach problems, coughs and colds. Oranges probably spread westwards across the globe thanks to sea traders. They are now produced on a large commercial scale in countries such as Israel and Brazil.

Sweet Orange essential oil has a gentle, soothing mental effect. It also helps to stimulate digestion and improve liver function, especially through abdomen massage. In 4 teaspoons carrier oil, add 4 drops Sweet Orange, 2 drops Lavender and 2 drops Peppermint. Stay out of direct sunlight for 12 hours after the massage as Sweet Orange can cause sun sensitivity.

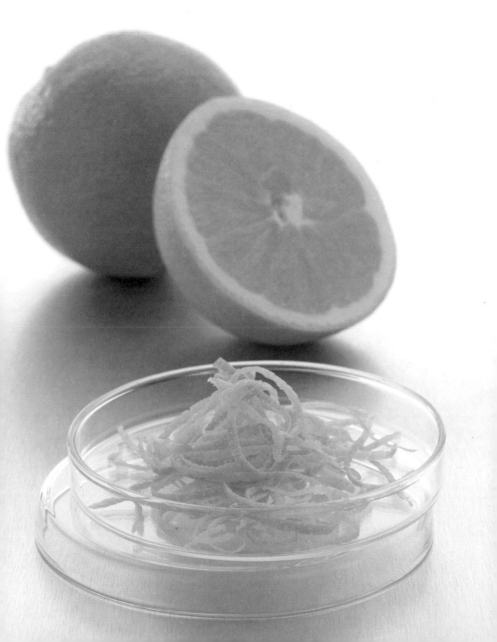

NEROLI [ORANGE BLOSSOM]
Citrus Aurantium

This exquisite aroma is taken from the blossoms of the Bitter Orange tree. These tiny creamy yellow flowers with golden centres have an astonishing fragrance; soft, sweet, slightly citrusy, yet rich, deep and musky. The flowers have to be collected by hand for distillation purposes, which is why Neroli is one of the most expensive essential oils along with Rose and Jasmine.

In early Renaissance times the story goes that an Italian princess of Nerola liked to perfume her gloves with orange flowers; the aroma became known as "Neroli". This trend spread to France where it became popular to perfume gloves with all kinds of flowers. Neroli essential oil also became one of the key ingredients in classic "eau de cologne", with Lavender, Rosemary, Orange peel and Orange leaf oils.

In aromatherapy, Neroli is regarded as one of the most effective stress-relieving essential oils; mentally it immediately diffuses anxiety, panic or feelings of shock, and physically it has been scientifically shown to relax heart palpitations. If you are expriencing panic or anxiety, which can cause the heart to race, try this special stress-relieving massage blend: in 4 teaspoons carrier oil, add 4 drops Neroli, 2 drops Sandalwood and 2 drops Frankincense for a wonderfully soft and uplifting aroma. Massage the blend over the upper back, shoulders and chest area.

Neroli is also one of the finest essential oils to use in skin care. It has a gently balancing effect on production of sebum, the skin's own natural lubricant; in more mature skins where dryness is often more pronounced, Neroli will soften and hydrate the upper skin layers, creating a peachy-soft texture. Neroli is non-allergenic and can help to improve the appearance of broken veins.

For a glorious after-shower body oil which is skin-soothing and deliciously perfumed: in 4 teaspoons carrier oil, add 4 drops Neroli and 4 drops Sweet Orange. Massage the blend carefully into your skin so that you are enveloped in the fragrance of orange trees — a truly wonderful way to beat the stress of the day.

LUXURY NEROLI SKIN FACIAL

For a clear complexion and softer skin, give yourself this special two-stage Neroli skin facial.

Neroli and Oatmeal Cleansing Scrub

Put 1 tablespoon fine oatmeal in a dish and add enough natural yoghurt to mix to a paste. Add 2 drops Neroli and mix. Apply to clean, make-up free skin, using small circles and avoiding the eye area. Rinse face and gently pat dry. The oatmeal and yoghurt are deep cleansing yet softening, and the Neroli soothes the skin.

Neroli, Jasmine and Frankincense Facial Oil

In 4 teaspoons deeply nourishing carrier oil (such as jojoba or apricot kernel), add 2 drops Neroli, 1 drop Jasmine and 1 drop Frankincense. Note the 1 percent formula (see page 47); facial skin is delicate and so requires less oil. Gently massage about ½ teaspoonful of blend over your face using small circles and avoiding the eye area. This recipe makes about eight applications.

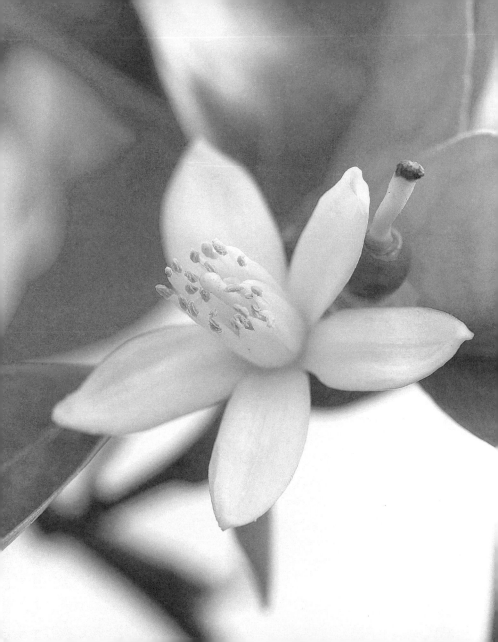

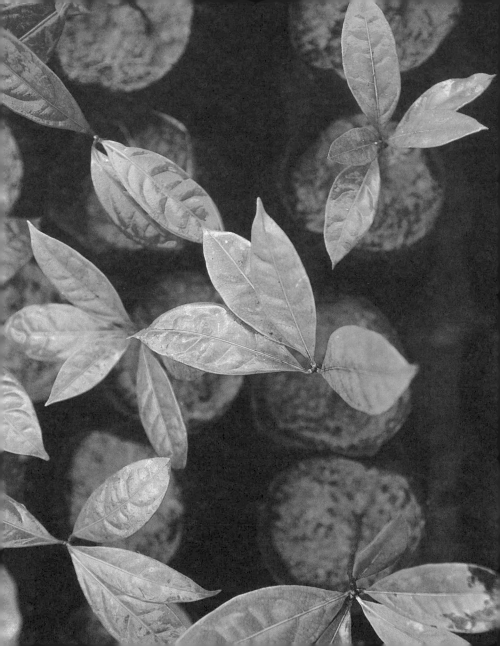

ROSEWOOD
Aniba Rosaeodora

Softly woody, sweet and fresh, the aroma of Rosewood is subtle and soothing to the senses. The oil is distilled from the wood of the tropical tree found mainly in Brazil and Paraguay. Brazilian Rosewood oil is often a by-product of deforestation, so try to buy oil from Paraguay, which is produced from sustainable sources.

Rosewood and Lavender complement each other aromatically and make an excellent destressing bath oil combination: try 3 drops of each in your bath water.

In skin-care, the oil is used extensively for soothing all skin types. For a nourishing and gently toning massage oil, in 4 teaspoons carrier oil, add 4 drops Rosewood, 2 drops Rose Absolute and 2 drops Myrtle. Rose soothes dryness and Myrtle deep cleanses the skin.

Rosewood also makes a soothing after-shave oil for men: in 4 teaspoons carrier oil, add 6 drops Rosewood and 4 drops Sandalwood. Both oils have an antiseptic effect, healing small cuts and calming shaving rashes.

ESSENTIAL OILS TO INSPIRE

The word "inspire" is derived from the Latin *spirare* (to breathe). Some fragrances automatically make you inhale deeply: imagine walking through a forest of evergreen trees and taking deep lungfuls of the resin-scented air. How does that make you feel? Perhaps incredibly light and wonderfully stimulated?

Many essential oils are obtained from woods and resins that have been used for thousands of years as incense. The calming, meditative effect they have on the mind is a prelude to attaining inner peace. Evidence suggests that the aroma of many types of incense can slow the rate of breathing. This aids the transition from a hectic pace of life to a more tranquil mental rhythm. In this state of mind we can receive inspiration.

Other pungent aromas help to open up the mind and stimulate creativity. These oils can help you study or improve your concentratation by arousing your mind – inspiring you to be creative and generate new ideas. All these oils work well in a vaporizer (see pages 38–9).

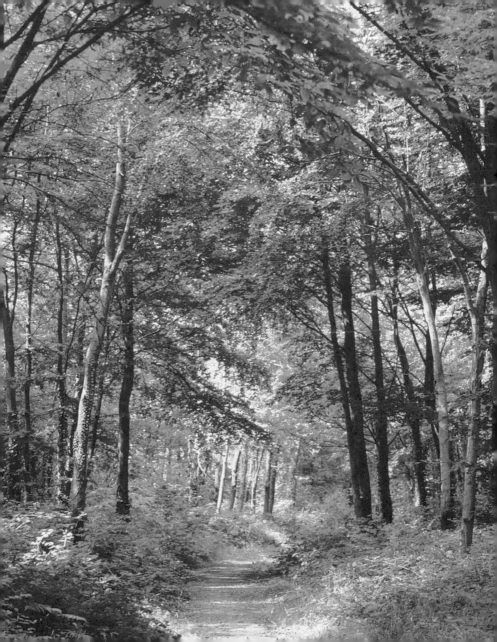

ATLAS CEDARWOOD
Cedrus Atlantica

Atlas cedarwood trees are originally from the Atlas Mountains of North Africa. These majestic, pyramid-shaped evergreens grow to more than 3om (100ft) tall. The essential oil is usually distilled from the branches and twigs of this reddish and highly aromatic wood.

In aromatherapy, Atlas Cedarwood is mostly used to help respiratory conditions. The vapour eases painful, chesty coughs and makes breathing easier. Using the inhalation method on page 40, add 3 drops Atlas Cedarwood and 3 drops Lavender to near-boiling water. Lavender also soothes the respiratory tract.

Atlas Cedarwood is great for restoring lacklustre hair and cleansing dandruff-prone scalps. In 4 teaspoons carrier oil, add 4 drops Atlas Cedarwood, 2 drops Frankincense and 2 drops Rosemary. Massage into dry hair, working from the scalp to the ends. Wrap your hair in clingfilm and cover with a towel for 20 minutes. Work a little shampoo directly into the hair, then rinse.

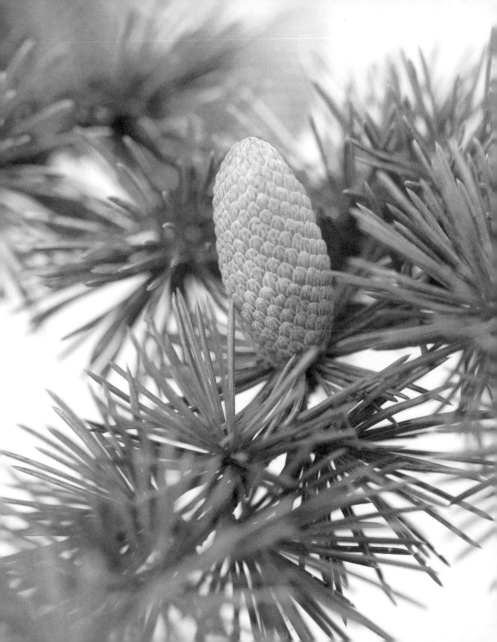

FRANKINCENSE
Boswellia Carteril

Woody, resiny, with a hint of spice and underlying sweetness, the aroma of pure Frankincense is instantly inspiring. Many people instinctively describe it as "ancient", recalling the peaceful interiors of sacred buildings, or the subtle aroma of fine wooden furniture. The fragrance encourages slow and steady breathing.

Frankincense trees come from Africa and parts of the Middle East, such as Oman. They are very slow growing, but can reach heights of up to 10m (30ft). They are not cultivated but grow wild in arid desert terrain, where they survive hostile conditions. If the tree's bark is cut or a branch falls away, to prevent moisture loss the tree immediately seals the gap with globules of pale yellow, sticky resin. It is these dried, highly aromatic grains or "tears" of Frankincense that are distilled to make essential oil.

The name "Frankincense" comes from two old French words, *franc* (meaning "true") and *encens* (meaning "incense"). The scent has been used in sacred rituals in Roman Catholic and Greek Orthodox churches for the past 2 millennia. Before that it was a key ingredient in ancient Egyptian ceremonies, used in embalming, medicines and cosmetics.

As valuable as gold or jewels, Frankincense has always been seen as a sign of wealth and status. The famous Egyptian Queen Cleopatra was so fond of it that she brought tree cuttings back to Egypt from the Middle East to plant in her private aromatic garden, so that the resin could be made into perfumes solely for her use.

In aromatherapy, Frankincense is used to heal damaged skin: cuts, minor wounds, grazes and spots are easily treated using a simple blend made up of 4 drops Frankincense and 4 drops skin-soothing Lavender in 4 teaspoons carrier oil. Using a cotton-wool pad, apply a small amount of the blend to the area twice daily.

In an inhalation treatment, Frankincense clears the chest and eases coughs; add 3 drops Frankincense and 3 drops cleansing Lemon to a bowl of near-boiling water, as described on page 40.

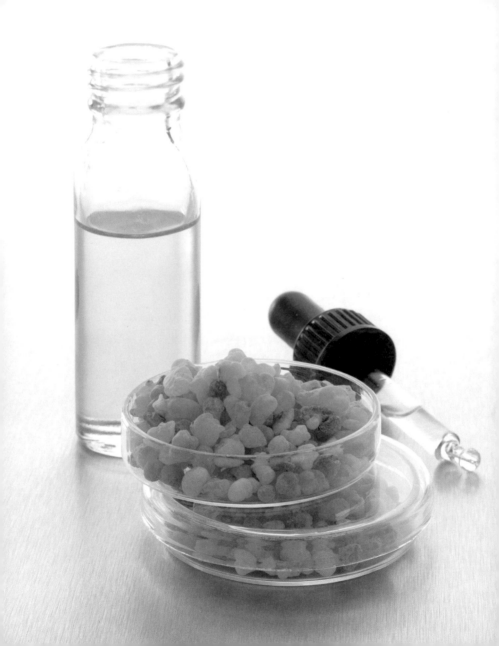

SPECIAL FRANKINCENSE FACE OIL

As a cosmetic and skin-enhancing essential oil, Frankincense is supreme. It encourages the normal replacement of surface skin cells, creating a soft and supple texture. It is particularly recommended for mature or dry skins which need extra nourishment, or to repair sun- and wind-damaged skin.

This exquisite facial treatment oil is soft and woody with sweet and rich floral notes. Use the blend nightly after thoroughly cleansing and toning your skin. In 4 teaspoons pure jojoba carrier oil, add 2 drops Frankincense, 1 drop Neroli and 1 drop Jasmine Absolute. Apply about ½ teaspoonful of the blend to your face using tiny circular movements. Start at the forehead and work down the face. Pure jojoba is a unique carrier oil because it resembles the oil the skin makes itself (sebum) and is therefore absorbed easily, leaving a silky texture. Frankincense and Neroli soften and replenish the skin, while Jasmine has a slightly toning effect. This amount will last about a week.

If we could see the miracle of a single flower clearly,
our whole life would change.

THE BUDDHA

(c.563–c483BCE)

Bread feeds the body indeed, but flowers feed
also the soul.

THE KORAN

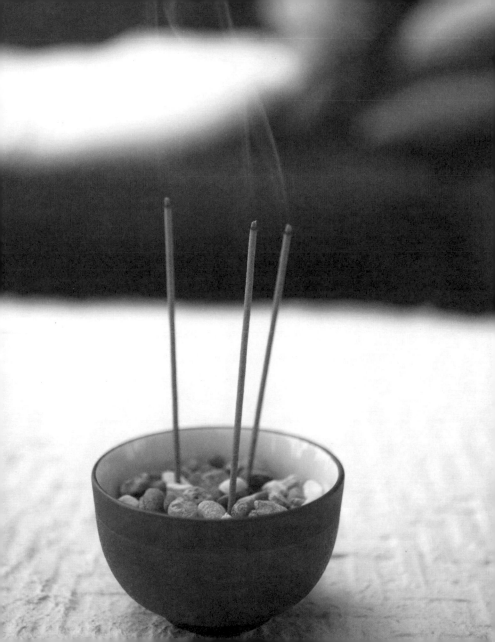

MYRTLE
Myrtus Communis

With eucalyptus-like notes and zesty undertones, Myrtle essential oil has a refreshingly fruity aroma. Small, dark green leaves and exquisite, creamy-white and gold flowers contrast with reddish bark on the branches and twigs. Native to the Mediterranean area, the sprigs of this evergreen shrub were burned as purifying incense in ancient Greece. Today, cleansing tea is made from the fresh leave in southern European countries.

The essential oil is distilled from the leaves and small twigs. If you have a cold, use 3 drops Myrtle and 3 drops antiseptic Tea Tree in a vaporizer to clear the air and improve breathing (see pages 38–9). The same oils can also be added to an inhalation treatment (see page 40), to open up the airways and ease breathing as well as loosen chesty congestion. In massage, Myrtle helps to energize tired, aching limbs. In 4 teaspoons carrier oil, add 4 drops Myrtle and 4 drops circulation-stimulating Rosemary. Massage into the legs after exercise.

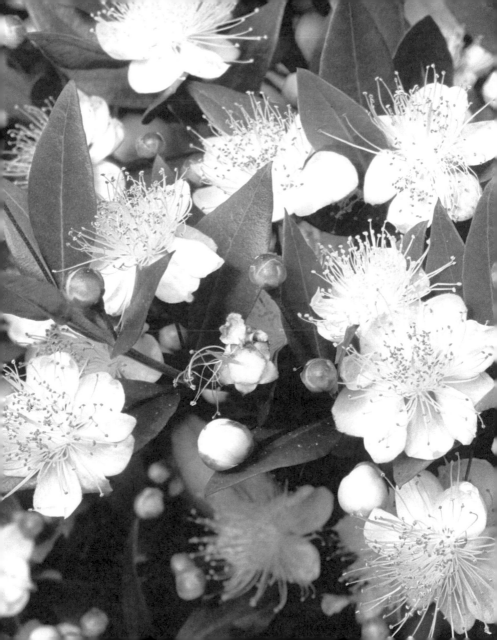

GRAPEFRUIT
Citrus X Paradisi

Pungent and bursting with freshness, grapefruit essential oil has a mouthwatering citrus aroma. It instantly clears the head of negative thoughts and instills a feeling of clarity. Squeezed from the peel of the fruit, the slightly golden yellow oil evaporates quickly, leaving a soft, citrus-tinged sweetness as an after-note.

Grapefruit trees are currently grown on a commercial scale in Florida, USA, Brazil and Israel; the essential oil is largely the by-product of the juicing industry. There is some uncertainty about how the grapefruit developed as a hybrid. One of its ancestors was probably the pumello fruit, brought by traders to the West Indies in the 1600s; cross-fertilization with orange trees is most likely to have produced the grapefruit.

The essential oil is rich in a limonene, which is regarded as highly cleansing to the system. It makes an excellent ingredient in aromatherapy blends created to help rid the body of toxins, especially toning up areas affected by cellulite, such as the thighs and bottom. A useful blend to try in 4 teaspoons carrier oil is 4 drops Grapefruit and 4 drops circulation-stimulating Rosemary. Massage daily into affected areas. Stay out of direct sunlight for 12 hours after the massage, as grapefruit can cause sun sensitivity.

Along with other citrus essential oils such as Orange and Lemon, Grapefruit is regarded as an antidepressant in aromatherapy, helping to encourage positivity and boost self-confidence. If you are suffering from anxiety or emotional upset, try massaging this zesty blend into your skin after a bath or shower: in 4 teaspoons carrier oil, add 4 drops cheering Grapefruit, 2 drops de-stressing Neroli and 2 drops strengthening Frankincense. The gently floral and fruity massage oil has a soft, woody undertone and is wonderfully comforting. Please observe the sun-sensitivity advice given above.

To refresh the air in your work space and clear your head, add 3 drops Grapefruit and 3 drops cleansing Peppermint to a vaporizer (see pages 38–9).

SPECIAL GRAPEFRUIT FOOT TREATMENT

We rarely pay enough attention to our feet, and yet they provide one of the easiest ways to give ourselves an aromatherapy treatment. Essential oils cleanse and deodorize the feet, while carrier oils nourish dry skin.

Grapefruit and Peppermint Foot Soak

Half fill a large plastic bowl with warm water and add 1 tablespoon purifying sea salt. Put 2 drops Grapefruit and 2 drops Peppermint into the water, and soak your feet for 15 minutes, making sure you can sit comfortably and relax. Pat the feet dry with a soft towel.

Reviving Grapefruit Foot Massage

In 4 teaspoons carrier oil, add 4 drops cleansing Grapefruit, 2 drops circulation-stimulating Peppermint and 2 drops warming Cardamom for a gorgeous, pungent yet fresh aroma. Massage about 1/2 teaspoon of blend into each foot to revive tired, aching feet and make them feel warm and tingly. This makes about four treatments.

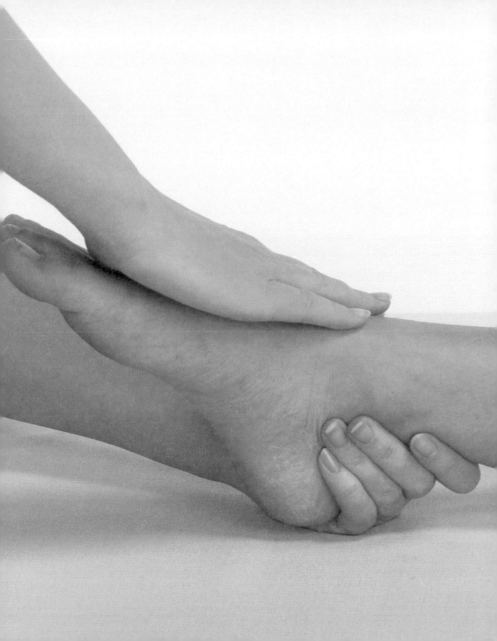

CARDAMOM
Elettaria Cardamomum

This spicy essential oil is warming and strengthening, with rich, tangy notes and a mouthwatering zestiness. In traditional Indian Ayurvedic medicine the whole spice and the essential oil are used to strengthen the immune system, ease chest infections and improve digestion. Cardamom pods are filled with tiny black, highly aromatic seeds – both the pods and seeds are distilled to yield the essential oil.

Cardamom makes a superb immune-boosting bath; if you feel the chills of an oncoming cold, add 2 drops Cardamom and 2 drops Tea Tree to your warm bath water and soak for at least 20 minutes. Then make a simple chest rub: in 4 teaspoons carrier oil, add 4 drops Cardamom, 2 drops cleansing Lemon and 2 drops anti-viral Tea Tree. Apply ½ teaspoon to the chest twice daily, to help fight infection. This blend can be used on children aged 3–10, but use half the stated number of drops of essential oil in the same amount of carrier oil.

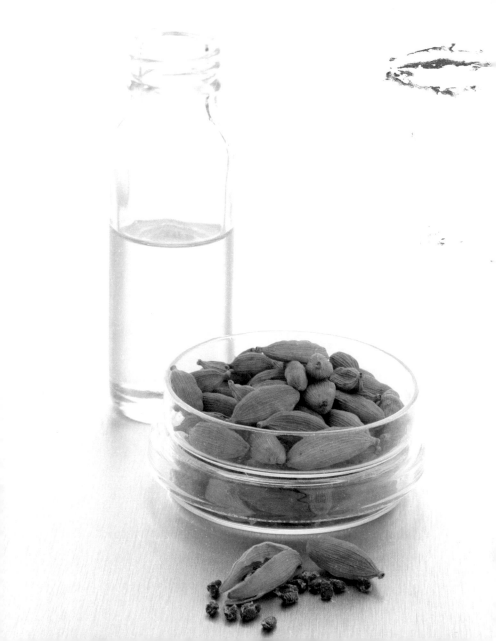

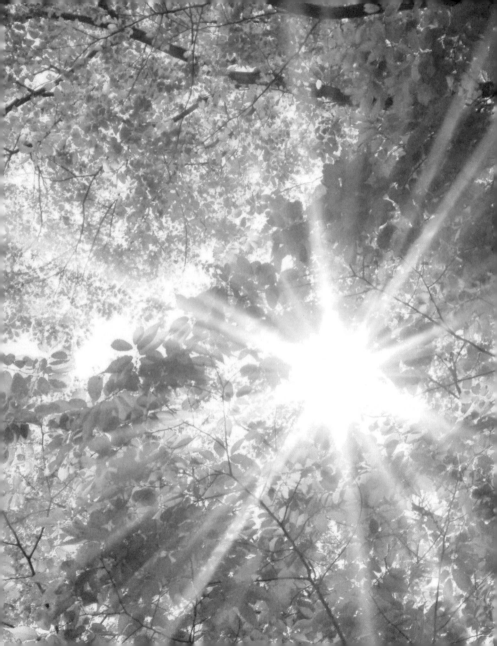

ESSENTIAL OILS TO LIFT THE SPIRITS

When something lifts the spirits, it produces a feeling of release — like light at the end of a tunnel, a sense of hope, a breath you take in which says "yes, wonderful". The idea that aromas can have that effect on us may be something new, but think about it — what about the smell of freshly baked bread, which can stop you in your tracks, make your mouth water and make you breathe deeply in appreciation?

In aromatherapy uplifting oils are vital because of their positive effect on the mind and their ability to shift feelings of anxiety and depression. The rich, delightful aromas of this group of oils can influence both moods and mental states, acting like shafts of light penetrating the grey fog of everyday weariness. The word "cheering" describes their effects perfectly: they refresh and restore the brain, bringing a sense of peace, calm and renewed focus. These oils have even been known to improve the mood of people with profound disabilities, showing the powerful effect of the sense of smell.

LEMON
Citrus Limonum

Delightfully fresh, clear and bright with sweeter, softer notes as it evaporates, Lemon instantly refreshes the atmosphere as soon as the aroma is released. It is a great essential oil to use in the workplace to cleanse the air: try using 3–4 drops in a vaporizer (see pages 38–9).

Lemon trees have large, dark green, shiny leaves and creamy-yellow flowers which turn into the bright yellow fruit. The best-quality oil comes from Sicilian lemons; the fruit is also cultivated in California and Florida. The oil is squeezed from the peel.

In aromatherapy, Lemon is regarded as cleansing and antiseptic: useful for treating colds or influenza. Try it as an inhalation (see page 40), using 3 drops Lemon and 3 drops anti-viral Tea Tree.

Lemon blends well with floral or inspiring oils to ease stress and anxiety. In 4 teaspoons carrier oil, add 4 drops Lemon, 2 drops Rose and 2 drops Frankincense. After massage, keep out of sunlight for 12 hours.

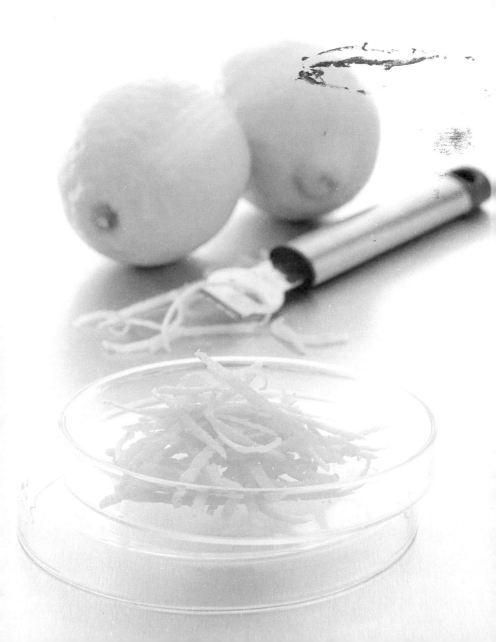

ROSE
Rosa Damascena, Rosa Centifolia

Two special kinds of rose yield beautiful fragrances for aromatherapeutic use. First there is the small damask rose (*Rosa damascena*), no more than 5cm (3in) across and with deep pink petals and a golden yellow centre. The rose has been cultivated for centuries in Turkey and parts of Eastern Europe as the main source of "Rose Otto", steam-distilled essential oil of rose petals.

Rose Otto has a sweet, honey-like aroma, with a faint hint of citrus. It is very labour-intensive to produce as the flowers have to be picked by hand and it takes about 200 blooms to release just one drop of essential oil. Some suppliers sell Rose Otto already diluted, as one or 2 drops in carrier oil, which is less expensive, but professional aromatherapists use the pure undiluted oil.

The second rose is another highly perfumed species called *Rosa centifolia*. It has larger, plumper blooms with many tightly packed petals. Grown commercially in Morocco and Turkey, it is chemically processed using solvents to obtain Rose Absolute. This has a different aroma, much heavier and sweeter with musk-like undertones. Rose Absolute is cheaper to buy than Rose Otto, but equally fine therapeutically. However, these two rose products are used differently in aromatherapy.

Rose Otto is used in massage blends to help emotional traumas such as grief, bereavement or deep emotional pain. Its subtle fragrance is gently enveloping and calming. Use 2 drops Rose Otto, 4 drops Mandarin and 2 drops Frankincense in 4 teaspoons carrier oil. Rose Otto is also used by professional aromatherapists to help repair inflamed, burned or damaged skin, and has even been clinically shown to help radiation burns.

Rose Absolute is extensively used in the formulation of natural creams and face-care products. It has a gently toning, yet soothing effect on the upper skin layers and helps improve the appearance of fine lines and broken veins. A face oil to try would be 2 drops Rose Absolute and 2 drops Jasmine in 4 teaspoons jojoba carrier oil. This blend nourishes mature or dry complexions and is highly recommended as a night-care treatment.

SPECIAL ROSE SKIN TREATS

These two special treats for the skin provide instant repair and smell heavenly. The skin soother helps to calm inflamed or angry skin (such as sunburn), while the facial oil is a nourishing and rejuvenating formula which helps dry, oily, combination or mature skins.

Rose, Lavender and Aloe Gel Skin Soother

Measure 4 teaspoons pure aloe vera gel (one of the best soothing agents to help calm and repair damaged skin) into a small, clean jar. Add 2 drops Rose Otto and 6 drops Lavender, stir and apply to sore areas as needed. This is a very useful formula to take on holiday.

Rose and Sandalwood Luxury Facial Oil

Using 4 teaspoons pure jojoba as a carrier oil, add 2 drops Rose Absolute and 2 drops Sandalwood. (Both of these ingredients are prized in India in perfumery as well as facial care.) This treatment can be used morning and night to enhance the complexion.

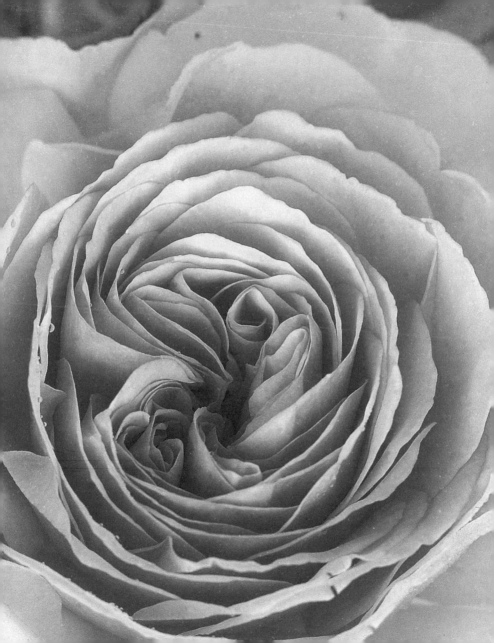

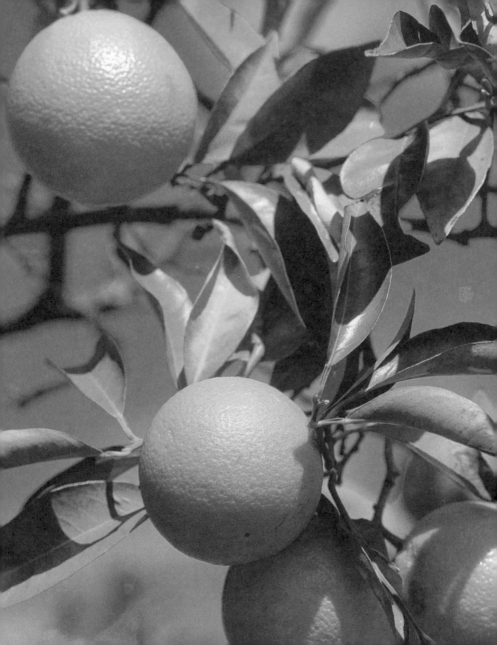

If seeds in the black earth can turn into
such beautiful roses, what might not the heart of man
become in its long journey toward the stars?

G.K. CHESTERTON

(1874–1936)

Cheerfulness is the very flower of health.

JAPANESE PROVERB

MANDARIN
Citrus Reticulata

Sweet, soft and full of zest, Mandarin is a cheering oil squeezed from the peel of this small, orange fruit. Its aroma is gentler than Grapefruit or Lemon. Mandarins originated in China and were brought to Europe in the 1700s, where they were successfully cultivated in Spain; South Africa and America are major producers today.

Mandarin has a sweet, innocent quality, making it ideal to use with children (aged 3-10): to help sleeping problems, try 3 drops Mandarin with 3 drops Lavender in a vaporizer (see pages 38–9). It also helps to alleviate stomach upsets and improve digestion: for abdomen massage try 2 drops Mandarin and 2 drops Peppermint in 4 teaspoons carrier oil. (Double the drops of essential oils for older children and adults.) Mandarin is also used to uplift negativity and ease depression. In 4 teaspoons carrier oil, add 2 drops Rose Otto and 6 drops Mandarin for a back, neck and shoulder massage. Avoid exposure to strong sunlight for 12 hours after the massage.

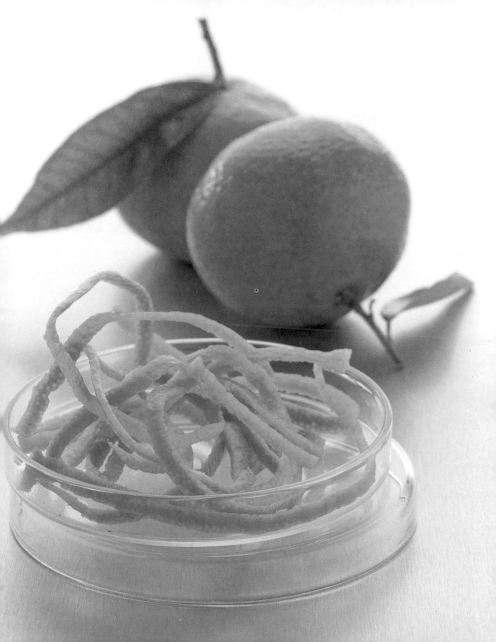

JASMINE
Jasminum Officinale

This exotic aroma is soft and sweet with hints of musk and rich, spicy undertones. It is a complex scent, and is often used in aromatherapy without other oils, simply because it stands alone as such a fine fragrance. The aroma is extracted from tiny, white, star-shaped flowers which bloom on delicate, climbing, dark green branches.

There are several different species; *Jasminum officinale* is commercially produced in Morocco and is the most commonly found variety in northern Europe. In India, a larger-bloomed species, *Jasminum grandiflorum*, is common, as well as the heavily scented *Jasminum sambac*. Branches of flowering jasmine are regularly made into garlands for Indian religious rituals – for example, to decorate statues of the gods, or to wear around the neck at weddings or other special occasions. For centuries, jasmine has also been prized in Far Eastern countries such as China, Nepal and Afghanistan, grown in the gardens of kings and potentates.

The flowers are far too delicate to be put through the intense heat of the distillation process, and so have to be chemically processed by soaking in cool solvent, which is then purified to create Jasmine Absolute. This concentrated aromatic liquid takes hundreds of thousands of tiny flowers to produce and is very expensive. However, a tiny amount goes a long way.

In aromatherapy, Jasmine Absolute is used to support deep emotional trauma, its rich, enveloping fragrance giving comfort, strength and reassurance at times when we feel vulnerable, lost and alone. It is particularly helpful for abdomen and back massage, to release physical tension which may have links to deep-rooted emotions. In 4 teaspoons carrier oil, use 2 drops Jasmine, 4 drops Sandalwood and 4 drops Rosewood for a deeply calming blend that is steadying to the nerves. Jasmine nourishes mature and dry complexions and slightly tones tiny veins under the surface, helping to improve local circulation. For a nourishing night facial oil: in 4 teaspoons jojoba oil, add 2 drops Jasmine and 2 drops skin-purifying Frankincense.

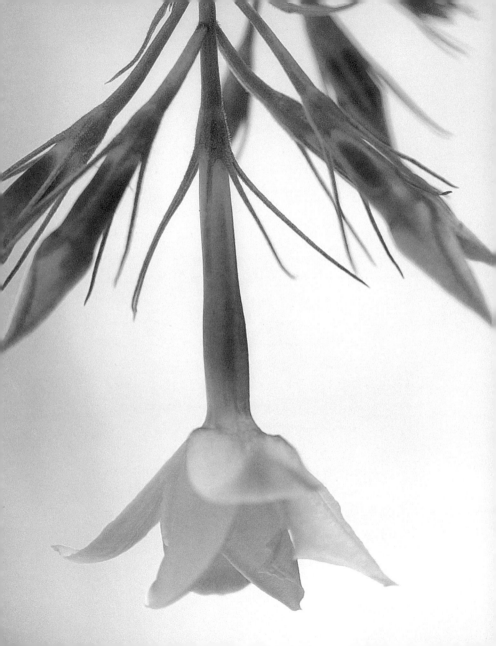

SPECIAL JASMINE PERFUME BLEND

Making a perfume using essential oils is actually very simple. Jojoba oil once again provides a perfect base because it has a waxy consistency and is compatible with the skin's own oils. It also keeps well, which is important, as a perfume blend is something you may want to use over a longer period of time, say 2–3 months.

Choosing essential oils for a perfume is extremely personal, but here is a combination using Jasmine Absolute which will give a lovely floral, fruity and woody aroma on the skin. In 4 teaspoons jojoba oil, add 2 drops Jasmine, 4 drops grounding Sandalwood and 4 drops uplifting Mandarin. Dab a tiny amount of perfume blend on the wrists and behind the ears. You will find the fragrance is very subtle and not as obvious as commercial perfumes, but bear in mind that you are using pure ingredients, whereas commercial perfumes are mostly made of synthetic chemicals. Once you get used to the subtlety of essential oils as a perfume you may find your fragrance preferences change.

YLANG YLANG
Cananga Odorata

The sweet, sensual, exotically floral aroma of Ylang Ylang makes it a favourite essential oil in aromatherapy, especially good for easing irritability and stress. Ylang ylang is a tropical tree with large, highly perfumed yellow and pink flowers. Native to south-east Asia, it is grown on a commercial scale in Madagascar, where the large flowers are steam distilled to release the essential oil.

Ylang Ylang is used in aromatherapy to calm and soothe the nervous system; it has been shown to alleviate emotional and physical stress, calming the heart rate. It can also help sleeping problems. First try a warm bath, using 2 drops Ylang Ylang and 4 drops Rosewood, then make a massage oil using 4 teaspoons carrier oil with 2 drops Ylang Ylang, 4 drops Mandarin and 2 drops Sandalwood, and massage the neck and shoulders.

Ylang Ylang's potent aroma can be overpowering to people who suffer from headaches or migraines. It is best to use 1–2 drops maximum with sensitive people.

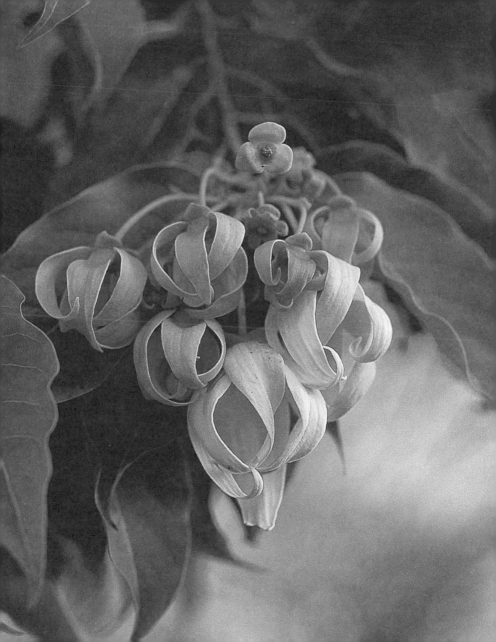

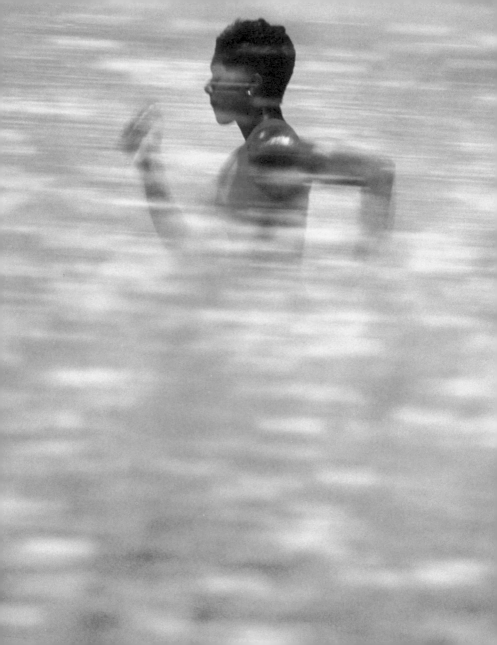

ESSENTIAL OILS TO REVITALIZE

This group of oils has powerful energizing properties, both on body and mind. They can improve circulation and bring a sensation of warmth or tingling to the skin when used in the bath or in massage. Many of them are preferred for sports massage, where muscles need deeper work to release stiffness, as they relieve pain and improve movement. They can also help with sluggish circulation, cold limbs or lack of physical energy.

Mentally these pungent fragrances have a bright and fortifying effect on the mind, clearing the thoughts and helping to improve concentration. They are useful in the workplace to help improve alertness, or in the car to keep focused while driving. Some people find them helpful after long-haul flights to keep awake and help the body avoid feeling jet-lagged.

Men are often more receptive to these pungent, powerful essential oils than to subtle aromas. This may be because these oils have a very marked physical effect, which men seem to appreciate.

PEPPERMINT
Mentha X Piperita

Bursting with the freshness of natural menthol, the penetrating aroma of peppermint brings a sense of clear-headedness, brightness and focus.

The plant is a vigorous annual herb with tough stalks and pointed, aromatic green leaves. It was a huge favourite of the Romans, who dressed their banqueting tables with it. In European herbal medicine peppermint tea is a classic remedy for stomach aches and headaches. In aromatherapy it is used in massage to aid indigestion and soothe muscular aches and pains. In 4 teaspoons carrier oil, add 2 drops Peppermint, 4 drops Lavender and 4 drops Black Pepper. Apply to the abdomen or aching limbs – you will feel the skin warming under your hands as you massage. To relieve headaches or migraine; in 1 teaspoon carrier oil, add 1 drop Peppermint, and massage into the forehead and neck. Peppermint is powerful, so very little is needed in blends with other oils to balance it. Avoid using on very sensitive skin.

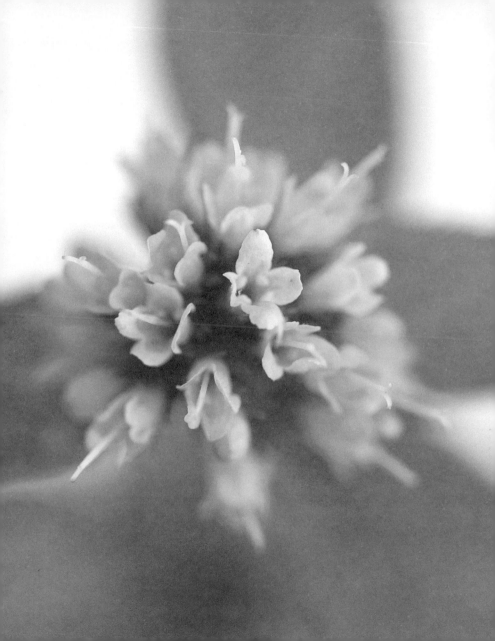

ROSEMARY
Rosmarinus Officinalis

The warm, pungent, almost fiery aroma of rosemary is instantly fortifying. It is an evergreen bush with highly aromatic dark green leaves. Each leaf has a matte velvety underside and a tougher shiny top side; the softer tissues below allow the plant to breathe, whereas the shinier surface filled with essential oil glands can withstand extreme temperatures and strong direct sunlight. Rosemary thrives in hot and dry conditions, growing in sandy soil where little else survives.

Native to the Mediterranean area, rosemary has been prized since ancient Greek times as a medicinal remedy. Hippocrates (5th century BCE), the father of modern medicine, used it to help liver and spleen disorders, and another famous Greek physician, Dioscorides (1st century CE), recommended it for diseases of the stomach by using it as a digestive herb, cooked with food. Branches of rosemary and juniper were burned as incense in ancient Greek temples.

Rosemary may well have been brought to Britain by the Romans. It became a popular culinary herb. In the 17th century the English herbalist Nicholas Culpeper recommended it for disorders such as dizziness, fainting fits or drowsiness. This was owing to the herb's powerful aroma, which he saw as fiery and stimulating.

With the development of more efficient distillation technology in Europe in the 16th and 17th centuries, rosemary became a popular fragrance, used in the making of "eau de cologne"; it was also a key ingredient in the formulation of "Hungary water", an alcohol-based liniment used to rub on aching limbs to improve the circulation and ease conditions such as gout.

In aromatherapy Rosemary is a vital circulation stimulant and muscle tonic. Used in massage, it warms the skin and eases stiffness and pain, bringing relief to aching muscles. In 4 teaspoons carrier oil, add 4 drops Rosemary, 2 drops Black Pepper and 2 drops Nutmeg. Note: Rosemary is not recommended for people with high blood pressure or anyone with epilepsy because of its powerful circulatory and brain-stimulating effects.

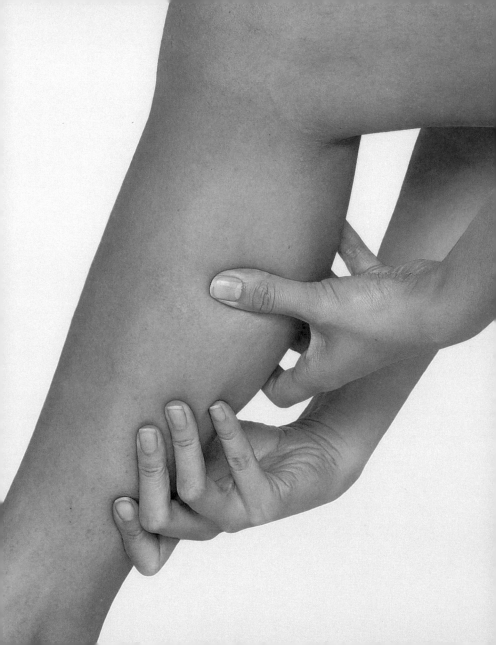

SPECIAL ROSEMARY FOOT AND LEG TREATMENT

This treatment is an excellent tonic for the feet and legs, especially after exercise or gardening, or standing all day. The bath treatment helps the circulation, while the massage releases tension, aches and pains.

Rosemary Bath Milk

Place 4 tablespoons of full-cream milk in a small bowl, and add 4 drops Rosemary. Run a warm bath (not too hot), and add the bath milk, stirring well. You can also add the leaves from a small sprig of fresh rosemary if you have any. Sit and soak for at least 20 minutes, making sure your legs are completely covered.

Rosemary Foot and Leg Massage Oil

In 4 teaspoons carrier oil, add 4 drops Rosemary, 2 drops Peppermint and 2 drops Lemon. Apply the blend to the feet, then work up the legs to the knees, using long, sweeping strokes. Your legs will feel alive and tingly.

To see the world in a grain of sand
And a heaven in a wild flower,
Hold infinity in the palm of your hand
And eternity in an hour.

WILLIAM BLAKE

(1757–1827)

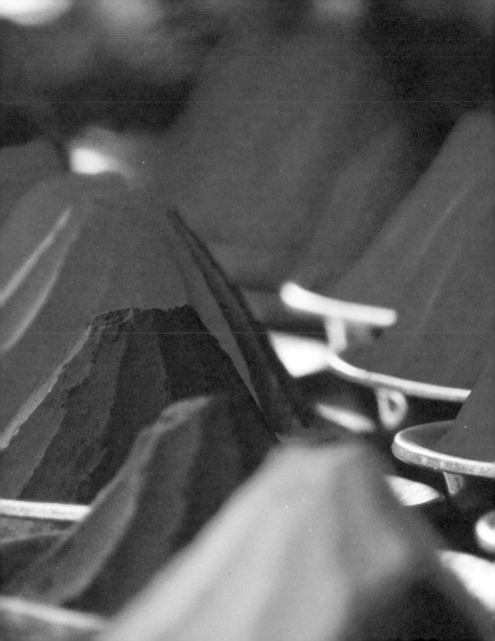

TEA TREE
Melaleuca Alternifolia

Green, fresh and cleansing, with a strong medicinal tone, Tea Tree is a vital ingredient in the aromatherapist's kit. Native to Australia, the essential oil is steam distilled from the extremely aromatic leaves of this evergreen tree, and has well-proven anti-bacterial, anti-fungal, antiseptic and anti-viral properties.

In aromatherapy Tea Tree is used as first-line defence against colds and flu. Combine with Lemon (use 3 drops of each) for an aromatic inhalation (see page 40). Or use it in a vaporizer (see pages 38–9) with other antiseptic oils such as Myrtle, to keep airborne germs at bay and help ease breathing: 3 drops of each oil in the unit will be effective for at least an hour.

Tea Tree also makes a wonderful aromatic chest rub for colds and coughs; in 4 teaspoons carrier oil, add 2 drops Tea Tree, 4 drops Atlas Cedarwood and 2 drops Lavender. Use morning and night to ease symptoms. Use half the number of drops for children aged 3–10.

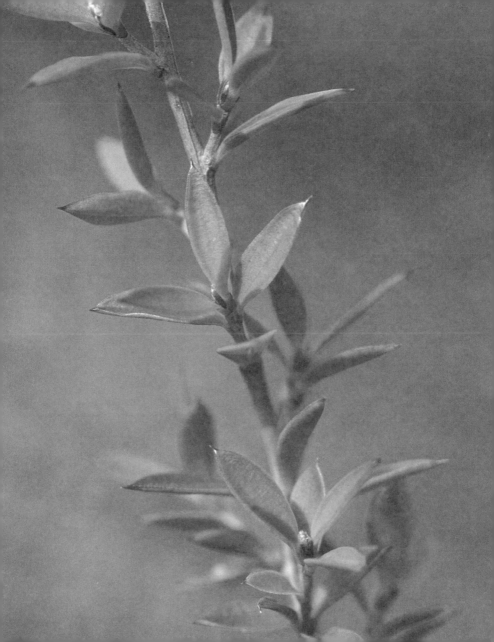

NUTMEG
Myristica Fragrans

Warm, spicy and penetrating with an initial strong sharp freshness, Nutmeg becomes sweet and soft as it evaporates. The oil is distilled from nutmegs, the fruit of the evergreen tropical tree. The outside husk, the mace, is removed and can be used as a spice, and the fruit themselves are dried and ground for use in cooking as one of the most popular flavourings. Nutmeg trees are native to Indonesia and continue to be cultivated there as well as in Sri Lanka.

Nutmegs were probably brought to Europe in the 1st century CE, by Arab traders journeying as far as Java and India. By the early middle ages (11th and 12th centuries), nutmegs were well-known and used to add spicy notes to both savoury and sweet dishes. However, only the very wealthy could afford them. In fact, spices such as nutmeg were considered so valuable that they were literally kept under lock and key; a housekeeper would carry the day's tally of spices in a locked box hanging from her belt. In the 16th and 17th centuries the trade in nutmegs became dominated first by the Portuguese and then the Dutch, who monopolized commercial routes to south-east Asia until the 19th century.

The traditional medicinal use of Nutmeg essential oil in south-east Asia is as a liniment to help aching limbs, stiffness and arthritis. It is a key ingredient in formulations such as Tiger Balm ointment, which is made for massaging into painful areas of the body. In Tibetan medicine nutmeg is regarded as an effective mental tonic and is used to help restlessness and depression. In early European herbal tradition it was regarded as a warming and comforting spice, helpful for protecting against negative moods and sleeplessness.

Nutmeg is used in aromatherapy to help emotional stress, tiredness or anxiety. It is powerful, so very little is needed. For a floral and spicy massage blend: in 4 teaspoons carrier oil, add 2 drops Nutmeg, 2 drops Neroli and 4 drops Lavender. To massage aching, tense muscles: in 4 teaspoons carrier oil, add 2 drops Nutmeg, 4 drops Rosemary and 2 drops Black Pepper.

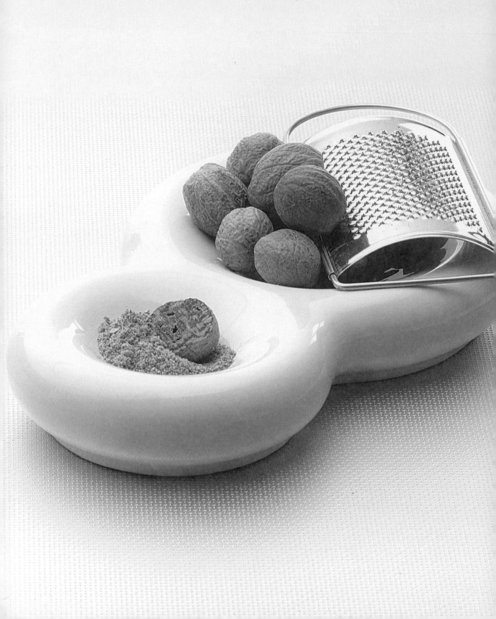

SPECIAL NUTMEG HAND TREATMENT

Cold hands affect people of all ages. This problem is caused by cold weather, but can also be stress-linked: when the body is tense, the circulation withdraws to the vital organs, away from the extremities. This hand treatment consists of a hot-water soak followed by a massage with warm carrier oil. It is also good for someone with mild arthritis in the hands, or symptoms such as repetitive strain injury.

First, prepare a massage blend using a small glass bottle: in 4 teaspoons carrier oil, add 2 drops Nutmeg, 2 drops Black Pepper and 4 drops Lavender. Put the bottle in a small bowl of very hot water to warm the blend while you soak your hands.

Fill another bowl with enough hot water to cover your hands. Add 1 drop Nutmeg and 1 drop Lavender to the water and soak your hands for about 15 minutes. Then dry them and massage in the warm blend; your hands will tingle and feel wonderfully energized. There is enough blend for two treatments.

BLACK PEPPER
Piper Nigrum

Spicy and pungent with soft, sweet undertones, Black Pepper essential oil is distilled from peppercorns, the dried fruit of a trailing vine with vibrant green leaves; it comes from Indonesia.

Black pepper has been used as a spice and remedy in India for thousands of years. It is a key ingredient in Indian Ayurvedic medicine, where its dry, warming properties make it vital for the massage treatment of colds, coughs and respiratory complaints; it is also used to support the immune system and aid digestion.

In aromatherapy, Black Pepper is used in massage to help poor circulation, cold hands and feet and aching muscles. In 4 teaspoons carrier oil, add 2 drops Black Pepper, 4 drops Cardamom and 2 drops Myrtle. Black Pepper also eases digestive troubles: in 4 teaspoons carrier oil, add 2 drops Black Pepper, 2 drops Peppermint and 4 drops Grapefruit. Apply to the abdomen, working in circles from right to left in a clockwise direction.

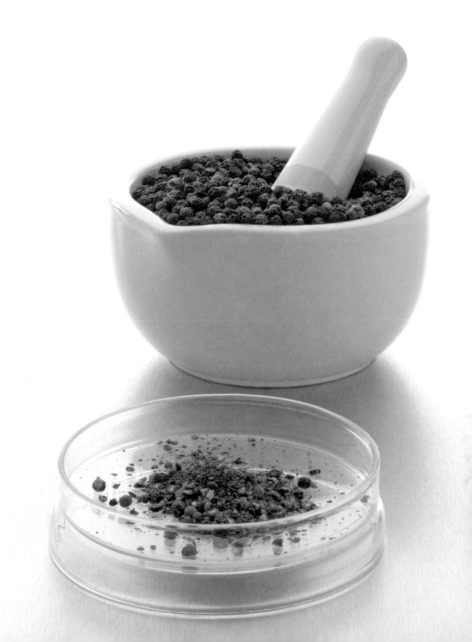

Once I have determined to move toward
enlightenment, even thought at times I might
become fatigued or distracted, streams of merit
pour down from the heavens.

SHANTIVEDA

(8TH CENTURY)

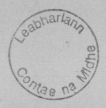

INDEX

Picture Credits

The publisher would like to thank the following people and photographic libraries for permission to reproduce their material. Every care has been taken to trace copyright holders. However, if we have omitted anyone we apologize and will, if informed, make corrections in any future edition.

Page 17 H.Kehrer/Zefa/Corbis; **20** Philip Craven/Robert Harding/Getty Images; **26** Marianne Majerus; **29** Masaaki Toyoura/Stone/Getty Images; **33** Julie Toy/Stone/Getty Images; **37** Phil Boorman/Photodisc Red/Getty Images; **40** Pierre Bourrier/Photonica /Getty Images; **49** Marianne Majerus; **53** Justin Pumfrey/Stone/Getty Images; **60** Botanica/Getty Images; **68** Edward Parker, Dorset; **71** Michael Busselle/Stone/Getty Images; **79** Trinette Reed/Photodisc Red/Getty Images; **81** Marianne Majerus; **88** DAJ/Getty Images; **95** Andrew Lawson Photography; **96** Marianne Majerus; **105** Deni Brown/OSF/Photo Library.Com; **106** Daniel Bosler/Stone/Getty Images; **115** David Sutherland/Photographer's Choice/Getty Images; **117** Dave Watts/NHPA; **124** J. Jaemsen/Zefa/Corbis